EXERCISES AT HOME TO LOSE WEIGHT

INCREASE YOUR MUSCLE MASS, TONE YOUR ABS, BICEPS, TRICEPS AND BUTTOCKS, TRAINING FOR WOMEN AND MEN

Jessy M. Brown

Copyright 2019© Jessy M. Brown

First Edition

Table of Contents

Introduction

It's a fact of modern life that most people don't get enough exercise.

This, coupled with a diet that is heavy on sugar and fast food loaded with fats, has led to a wave of overweight and obese people in most Western countries, a tidal wave that is becoming increasingly difficult to reverse.

The problem is that, for most people, it's too easy and convenient not to exercise.

If you need the basics of everyday life - even if it's just a carton of milk or a loaf of bread - it's faster and more convenient to get in the car and drive to the store than to walk.

If you have to reach the third or fourth floor when you go to the office, it is easier (though not always faster) to take the elevator instead of the stairs.

However, many people are willing to pay hundreds or even thousands of dollars each year to be a member of a gym or a fashionable fitness club in order to stay in shape.

This doesn't make much sense, so this book is here to tell you that it doesn't have to be that way.

I'm going to teach you to put your money in your pocket and exercise in a natural way, in a way you don't even realize.

Humanity survived for thousands of years before anyone came up with the idea of "exercising in the gym.

Of course, modern man's life expectancy has increased significantly over the past two hundred years, but I suspect this has little to do with the proliferation of luxury gyms and expensive gyms.

The good news is that exercise can be done naturally every day. With a little thought, it's not hard to think of many opportunities to exercise without having to resort to spending the money earned on gym fees.

Let's start by seeing why exercise is so important in modern life.

Why is exercise so important?

For most people, drinking or exercising tends to be reactive.

That is, there has to be something going on in your life that forces you to re-evaluate what you are doing. Something happens that makes them realize that they need more exercise as a way to change the things that go wrong in their lives.

For example, many people reach a point in their lives when they finally recognize what they have known for a long time, that they are overweight or obese. Perhaps most importantly, after finally accepting that their weight really is a problem, they make a conscious decision to do something about it. Therefore, they make a weight loss diet of some description and, for most people, exercising is part of the weight loss process.

The saddest part is that if such overweight or obese people had regulated their calorie intake and exercised regularly beforehand, they would never have reached the state that requires such drastic action.

Others may decide to start exercising in an effort to slow the aging process, often at a time in their lives when they finally understand that the arrival of the reaper's death is much closer than they once imagined.

This is good, but it's also a classic "better late than never" case. The fact is that if people who exercise late in life had done so only twenty or thirty years earlier, their efforts to delay the inevitable would have been more effective.

That's the point about exercise that a lot of people ignore. Exercise should not be something that is done reactively, at a point where it has to be done in an attempt to reverse something that has already happened.

Exercise should be seen as a proactive step that everyone can afford as one of the best preventive measures they can take.

Increased physical activity will increase your heart rate and strengthen all the muscles in your body. The heart is just one muscle and all muscles are strengthened the more often they are worked.

This resulting increase in heart activity will automatically speed up blood circulation through your body, which in turn will deliver more oxygen and nutrients to all of your organs.

Regular exercise helps increase the lungs' ability to absorb and use oxygen, is effective in reducing body fat, and lowers levels of sugars and "bad" cholesterol in the blood.

A regular exercise program (if started early enough) can also help delay the inevitable aging process.

Exercise will strengthen the body, making it more resistant to disease and injury.

Exercising regularly also improves your overall quality of life. It makes you feel better physically and mentally.

It allows you to enjoy everything you do much more than you did before, because you have increased your energy and vitality and that allows you to become more involved in everything that is happening.

All of these are benefits you can enjoy by simply starting exercising now, rather than waiting until you 'have to' for one reason or another.

So, am I advocating enrolling in one of the "luxury fitness clubs" mentioned above or enrolling (and paying for it) in an expensive gym? Absolutely not!

There are dozens of opportunities to "exercise" during the course of the average day, and it's really just a matter of making the right decisions, as you'll see.

In some parts of the world, exercise is a natural part of life, because people in many places simply do not have the choices that those living in the rich countries of the West have.

For example, they don't eat hamburgers or chips every other day, because there is no fast food store in the local mall (in fact, there is no local mall).

They don't get in the car to go everywhere, because they don't have a car, and as there are no buses, they go everywhere.

These people are forced to adopt a lifestyle that in many respects is healthier than the one that most people in developed Western countries are accustomed to because they have no other choice.

You have a choice, and it's up to you to choose to live in a way that benefits you and your health, rather than harming it.

Part of that choice is to exercise regularly, and the sooner you start working your body a little bit more than you do now, the better it will be.

> ***Some precautions***

Exercise is good for you, but you need to make sure you're able to handle whatever you plan to do before you start.

Especially if you haven't exercised regularly for a while, it makes sense to get a full physical before starting any exercise regimen.

Tell your doctor why you are undergoing the checkup and what you plan to do, because you may have some advice or input to help you streamline your plans.

Also understand that most people who have not exercised for some time should start slowly, no matter what form of exercise they plan to follow.

Trying to do too much, too quickly could be potentially more harmful than doing nothing at all, because the stress you exert on your body can be too much. The risk of injury or even worse is much greater if you try to do things too quickly.

Another thing you should do before starting any exercise regimen is to recognize and accept your age and general physical condition.

Although we all like to believe that we can still do things that we could do in our teens and twenties, when you get to the second half of your life the truth is that you simply can't do what you could at any given time.

Accept it and try to avoid seeing it as a challenge to be overcome. Doing so will probably lead you to try to do too much, and again, that can significantly increase the risk of injury.

Injury is one of the safest ways to stop your dry exercise program, so the greater risk inherent in doing too much too soon isn't worth it.

Walking is the first thing you should do

When was the last time you walked anywhere?

I'm not talking about hiking in the mountains and walking into deep valleys. I don't mean road marches either.

Think about it. When was the last time you made the effort to walk, instead of jumping in the car or the subway?

Walking is one of the easiest and most effective forms of aerobic exercise (exercise that increases heart rate and therefore blood circulation) that exists and is something that is available to everyone at no cost.

In fact, walking will save you money and help you protect the world we live in.

It saves money on your gas bill and reduces the amount of pollutants generated by the car that are pumped into the atmosphere we all breathe, for example.

Walking regularly helps reduce the risk of heart disease, osteoporosis, and some types of cancer, as well as reduce body fat and blood pressure. Unlike many other forms of exercise (e.g., jogging), walking is low-impact and low-intensity, so the risk of injury is also minimized.

If you walk a couple of miles to the store instead of taking the bus or the subway, then you do yourself a favor, plus save a dollar or two in your pocket.

Walking is something you can do anytime, anywhere and at absolutely zero cost. All you need is a pair of comfortable shoes, preferably with padded soles to protect your feet and the leather upper (or other natural materials such as canvas) that will allow you to breathe.

Many modern sports shoes are constructed entirely of synthetic materials (usually some form of plastic) and therefore wearing them leads to an unhealthy accumulation of sweat. This can lead to fungal conditions such as an athlete's foot, and having such a condition would seriously reduce your exercise program, so wearing the right shoes from the start is extremely important.

Maybe you think you don't have time or a chance to walk? Let me tell you, that's just an excuse.

Everyone has the opportunity to walk if they are willing to make small adjustments in the way they live their daily lives.

For example, if you take public transportation to work every day - the subway or the bus - how about getting off a couple of stops early and walking down the street?

the rest of the way? You'll add five minutes to your travel time, but if that can add a couple more years to your life, wouldn't you consider that a reasonable compensation?

Have you ever thought about taking kids to school, instead of piling them up in the back of the truck and driving them the mile you take? Not only would walking be good for you, but it also teaches your children good habits from an early age, and there is research indicating that children who are taught that walking is a good idea when they are young tend to continue to do so throughout their later life.

You protect your own health and that of your children for years with only a small change in your daily routine.

How about we take the dog for a walk in the morning and one more time, last thing at night?

Don't you have a dog? You don't need a pedigree dog, so go to the local dog rescue centre or shelter and find a new four-legged friend.

Walking the dog in this way may mean getting out of bed ten minutes earlier, but, as I suggested earlier, isn't that a reasonable compensation for a few more years?

Sometimes, no matter how good your intentions, you'll have to use the car. If, for example, you work in a remote location without adequate public transportation, or need to go to the local mall to do a full week's shopping, then you probably have no choice but to drive.

In this situation, what if you park your car in the car park at the furthest point from your destination and walk a few hundred metres?

If you're shopping, you're going to push a cart with all your groceries from the store to your car, so that adds a little extra effort (i.e., exercise) to what you're doing, and if you're working, then you're not going to wear anything heavy every day, so there's no excuse not to do this!

How long should I walk?

The answer to that question is: the more you walk, the better and the more your health will benefit.

At first, at least, take it easy with short ten-minute walks. Start each walk relatively slowly and smoothly, accelerating in the middle, and end with a brief "cool down" when you go for a walk.

Gradually (but not too gradually) increase this to walking at least 30 minutes a day at least five times a week, although it is not necessary for you to exercise for the full thirty minutes of the session. Three of ten minutes

Walking would, for example, be equally effective, so if that fits better with your daily routine, then that's the way to go.

However, you should also keep in mind that thirty minutes a day, five times a week, is the minimum time you should devote to walking, not your ultimate goal. If you can drive one hour a day, that's even better!

If you're serious about your walks (and remember that we're talking about your health and well-being, so you should), you may want to invest in a pedometer with which you can count the number of steps you take each day.

Use it to establish how many steps you take on a normal day and then try to increase that number by at least 2,000 more steps as your initial goal.

At a fast pace, that represents a couple of extra miles a day, so it's a good start, but this should be considered as a start only. Try to increase this figure as much as you can and your health will inevitably benefit from your efforts.

It is natural that there are times when you are less motivated than others to take your walk. This is when having a dog to exercise with can be a great motivator, or taking children for a walk would serve a similar purpose.

Otherwise, walking can also be a very sociable form of exercise, so what if you try to gather a group of friends or work colleagues to go for a walk together?

Some of those people are probably

paying hundreds of dollars in gym membership dues right now, and if you can show them how they can get exactly the same exercise benefits for free, then they are more than likely to accept your challenge.

Stairs: Everything you need

Forget the elevator!

Many people, especially those living in congested cities, work in office towers. They use the elevator every day of their lives to get from the ground floor to the floor where their office is located.

Others use elevators in department stores, apartment towers, etc.

Forget the elevator and take the stairs, because climbing stairs is one of the most effective forms of aerobic exercise you can do.

This was clearly proven by a British study about ten years ago, when researchers discovered that for moderately sedentary people, only a few minutes climbing stairs every day demonstrably improved their cardiovascular health.

This study was of particular interest because it supported the idea that taking several short jets of exercise every day will make a significant difference in your health (hence the idea that you can walk ten minutes a day three times, rather than just one thirty-minute session).

The study required 20 college-aged women living relatively sedentary lives to climb 200 steps in less than two-and-a-half minutes.

This represented a "fast but

comfortable" rhythm according to the researchers who conducted the study, but the first time they did so, it served to trigger the heart rhythms of the test subjects up to about 90% of the anticipated maximum heart rhythms.

Despite this, the test subjects went from making one promotion per day during the first week to six per day in the sixth and seventh weeks.

Therefore, this meant that the test subjects were climbing stairs for about thirteen and a half minutes a day at the end of the test, which (if the point is unclear) represents less than a reasonably rigorous quarter of an hour of exercise each day.

At the end of this relatively modest (and completely free) exercise program, the women tested were much better prepared than before. All indicators have improved considerably. Their heart rate immediately after the ascent had slowed noticeably and their breathing had also slowed, indicating that they needed less oxygen to "feed" their efforts.

On the other hand, their HDL levels had increased, which is good, because high-density lipoprotein is also sometimes referred to as "good" cholesterol. High levels of HDL in the blood appear to play a role in reducing the risk of heart attack, while low levels appear to do the opposite by increasing the risk of heart disease.

It is clear how effective it can be to climb the stairs as an exercise, and even more so if you climb the stairs in pairs.

This significantly increases the work that

the leg muscles have to do, and that in itself increases the aerobic effects of your exercise to a remarkable degree.

All this proves one thing.

You don't have to exercise for hours to enjoy the benefits an 'exercise' will bring you. Less than 15 minutes of climbing stairs a day will significantly improve your overall aerobic health and will cost you nothing at all.

So the next time you go to the office or the store and are tempted to enter a full, hot, sweaty elevator, think about it for a moment.

Make the most of your house and garden

In the final analysis, exercise is nothing more than making your body work, burning energy using your muscles to achieve certain goals you set for yourself.

In times past, when physical work was much more common and important, man did not really need to worry about what is essentially an artificial requirement as a way of burning energy.

Today, the Western lifestyle in general involves very little physical work based on work, hence the need to think of ways to exercise.

Running a house and a home requires work and effort, however, whether you realize it or not, you're exercising every time you try any kind of chores around the house.

For example, many women would find vacuuming and dusting the house tedious and tedious. Cleaning windows, ironing and washing clothes probably wouldn't be one of the funniest activities either.

However, all of these activities represent an exercise you don't even know you're doing, as evidenced by the fact that 15 minutes of vacuuming and dusting burn an additional 40 kilocalories for a 40-year-old woman who weighs 78 kilos and measures 165 centimeters.

That's not a huge amount, but it indicates that you're working, and therefore you're doing a kind of exercise, even without realizing it.

Mowing the lawn, digging in the garden and weeding will have an equally beneficial effect, with fifteen minutes of doing this type of activity burning more than fifty calories for the same woman.

Since "gardening" is an activity that many people enjoy and spend many hours involved in, there is the potential for serious exercise. I suspect that most people would never consider this an exercise, so that makes it much easier to do.

Is the car dirty? If so, forget about the idea of taking it to the car wash, because washing your hands yourself has many benefits. Not only will you save the money you would otherwise have spent on car washing and do your bit to help the environment, but you'll also be able to stretch, as you'll have to reach the roof of the car, bend and work your muscles. These are muscles that are generally not used if working in a sedentary office environment.

In the case of washing the car, even at a gentle and pleasant pace - after all, it's not a race - you'll still burn 150 kilocalories per hour.

Do you have children or does a family member who lives relatively close to you have a family? Do them a favor by taking the kids to the park for a smooth game of whatever you want - soccer, baseball, cricket, tennis - it doesn't really matter what sport it is.

The point is that it is good for all of you both physically and spiritually, it costs nothing and will give you a great appetite.

You want to move faster?

Maybe walking isn't for you, so here's an alternative.

Next time you get in the car, point to the bike shop and buy a bicycle.

As a method of getting from point A to point B, cycling has almost everything in its favor and very few drawbacks.

To begin with, cycling is a great exercise, as well as being challenging, sociable and a lot of fun.

It is environmentally friendly - no pollutants are emitted when using the power of the pedals - uses all the major muscle groups of the lower half of the body, and gives your heart an excellent workout as well.

For many people who cannot do other sports such as jogging due to the impact and pressure this sport exerts on their joints, cycling is ideal.

Because the bike supports most of the weight of your body, the impact on your joints is significantly reduced while you are on your bike, so cycling is something that almost anyone can do.

It burns calories and helps reduce the levels of fat in your body as well, so if you are interested in losing weight while having fun, cycling would definitely be a sport to consider.

Another advantage of cycling is that most of us can already do it, so no additional special training is required. This can be an advantage compared to other forms of exercise in which training is needed, because the very idea of going through a training program can discourage you from getting involved in the first place. However, once you know how to ride a bicycle, it is a case of, once learned, never forgotten.

If you want to get started in cycling, the first tip is that, as with all forms of exercise, you should start slowly, especially if you haven't done any exercise in the recent past (and that condition applies to a large number of people!).

The next thing you have to do is decide what kind of bike you want. There are many different types available, such as racing road bikes, touring bikes and mountain bikes.

What do you plan to do on your bike and where do you want to ride it? Answer that question, and it will tell you which type of bike is best for you.

Not everyone has access to the same facilities and resources or will use their bicycles for the same purposes, because these factors vary from country to country and sometimes from area to area.

For example, not everyone is cycling on the roads, because one of the few disadvantages of cycling is that it can be quite dangerous to do so in many places, because the level of driving of cars and drivers varies greatly.

In some countries (the UK is a great example) there are an increasing number of bicycle lanes in some of the most beautiful areas of the countryside, so you may decide to cycle off-road if you have access to these resources and facilities. This will, of course, indicate the direction of a mountain bike instead of a road racing machine.

In Japan, it is common to see a mother taking two kindergarteners to school by bicycle. In this situation, a city bike is the best option.

Therefore, everyone will choose their bike according to their specific needs, so try to establish which are yours before investing in a bike.

Don't be too proud to take a look at second-hand stores when you're looking for a bike either. You'll find some amazing bargains, and (like an avid second-hand store browser) it's amazing that almost every store I've ever visited seems to have bikes almost permanently in stock! Also, try online resources like Overstock, where you can buy new bikes at factory prices, as well as auction sites like eBay.

Once you have decided on cycling, you should invest in basic equipment, such as an approved safety helmet and lights suitable for your machine (both front and rear).

Carrying a basic set of tools and a spare air chamber (which you should know how to change) is a good idea, and wearing bright, reflective clothing will help you stay safe, no matter where you're riding your bike.

At first, keep riding on a reasonably flat terrain until you have built up resistance and endurance, and be prepared for very stiff legs the day after your first couple of rides. That tells you that you're working muscles that haven't been used for some time, so it's a good thing even if it doesn't feel that way at the time!

Once you have built from this starting point, then start including hills and inclines in the cycling routes you have chosen, as this will increase the work you have to do while pedaling, and that considerably increases the aerobic benefits of your cycling training.

As mentioned at the beginning of this section, cycling can be a very sociable pastime, and if you want to enjoy your cycling more, why not join a local cycling club? There are many online resources where you can find information about these groups, such as Cycling England, Bicycle Tours USA and Cycling News.

In addition, there are sites that offer a lot of general cycling guidance and help, such as the About.com cycling page and Why Cycle, which is a UK-based site that is full of good advice and ideas that can be used when you pedal anywhere.

Submerge!

Another excellent low-impact sport that almost everyone can practice is swimming.

Swimming is a great exercise that puts a minimum of stress on your body while working all the major muscle groups throughout your body.

Because your body weight is always fully supported by the water while you are swimming, it is a form of exercise that literally has no impact on your joints, making it quite ideal for anyone.

It's a sport that requires only the most basic equipment - a bathing suit (obviously!) plus glasses to improve your underwater vision and protect your eyes. Some people also prefer to wear earplugs while swimming (especially those who are susceptible to ear infections) although this is not strictly necessary.

Swimming is an excellent complete aerobic exercise, since it works all the muscles of the body. The more "blows" of swimming (for example, blows to the chest, back, etc.) you know, the more benefits you will get from swimming. This is because the different actions required for each stroke naturally require different muscle groups for successful application.

To get all the benefits of swimming you need to know how to swim, but it's never too late to start learning.

Most local swimming pools offer lessons

for everyone, from the youngest babies to adults, so it shouldn't be too hard to find a place where you can learn and don't be embarrassed to join the class.

You certainly won't be alone, though, if you're the type who can be shy about this sort of thing, then it should be possible to receive private tuition.

Make an effort to set aside time each week when you can go swimming, and go with your friends or (better yet) your children, as this will increase the fun of what you are doing considerably. The more fun it is, the less it looks like a real exercise.

As always, start slowly, because although swimming is the mildest sport in terms of the negative impact of the "shock" it will have on your body (there is none), it is still exhausting. Your heart will be getting serious training when you're swimming, although you probably won't realize the fact, so don't try to do too much and too fast.

Once you have the fundamentals in place - at least you can swim - then to get the maximum benefit from your new skill, you should consider putting some kind of plan in place.

Otherwise, it's too easy to get into a routine, doing the same number of pool lengths every day, and that can become tedious very quickly. When you do, you may start to lose interest, go less and less to the pool and it won't be long before you stop going completely. And then you start all over again, without any exercise.

Here's a general plan for getting the

most out of swimming. This plan will seriously increase your fitness levels in two four-week periods. Each of these four weeks consists of three weeks of active swimming training followed by a week of recovery and relaxation.

If that sounds immediately frightening or troubling, don't be alarmed. This is not a program for those who are planning to become Olympic class swimmers! However, it is designed to be a program that will bring noticeable increases in fitness levels as soon as possible, so, if that's the main goal of exercise, then this is ideal for you.

The fundamentals of this plan are essentially the same, however, many times you will be swimming, as well as the goals. What you're going to do is improve your fitness while learning better swimming techniques, so you can swim more efficiently.

This is important, because getting stronger while still applying a poor technique is not really going to help you. Although the main goal is to get fit through exercise, improving your swimming skills is also a central point of this plan.

In practical terms, technique and aptitude go hand in hand, in the sense that you can't maximize one without focusing on the other. On the other hand, it's quite impossible to focus on both at the same time, and that can lead to frustration and the feeling that you're not getting better or that you're not getting anywhere.

Therefore, this program mixes the development of swimming skills and exercise, but not at the same time.

It's a training plan that focuses primarily on meeting your overall need to improve overall fitness levels, but it's still a training plan that's highly adaptable. In other words, if your long-term goal or goal goes beyond simply getting a little more fit, then you can modify this plan to suit your specific needs.

For example, if you're looking for nothing more than good aerobic training, then this plan will work for you just the way it is, because running through the plan just once will dramatically increase your fitness levels.

If you then want to take your fitness to the next level, simply repeat the program and keep doing it until you reach the point where you are happy.

on your condition. So it's just a case of maintaining that condition with regular swimming sessions.

This is a systematic plan, so you need to have a pencil and paper to write things down. Some calculations are also needed, so a calculator can also be useful. Alternatively, type everything into your computer in a Word document, and also use the built-in calculator.

In the first week of four, each training session should last 45 minutes. Of these, spend the first 9 minutes warming up with a little gentle stretching by the pool, followed by a little moderate swimming. Spend the next nine minutes on your swimming technique, followed by twenty-two minutes of your main period of physical training. In this period, swim fast for thirty seconds, followed by 30 seconds at medium pace, another thirty seconds fast and then thirty seconds rest. This is repeated until the period is over. Finally, there is a five-minute cooling period of gentle swimming.

Over the next three weeks, increase the "main" training period by 5-10% per week. This is not at the expense of any of the other sessions, so your total pool time should increase over the weeks.

Decide how many swimming sessions you can do per week and stick to that plan. Be as consistent as you can, so if you do five sessions in the first week, try to do the same (or as close as you can) every week.

Also, if possible, try to increase your

"main" training period in each session. If, for example, you are planning a total increase of 10% during the week and have five sessions written down, start with a 5% increase, then 6% in the next session, 7% in the next and so on.

Even at the end of the total eight-week cycle, you should not swim more than 75 minutes per session in total, and I do not recommend that you increase your core workout by more than 10% in any given week. A target increase of five to ten minutes per week of "main" training is a good target.

Be sure to complete each 'section' of each training session, and be sure to rest up to one minute between each 'section' of the session.

In each section of your training

sessions, do everything as many times as you can, so you don't miss any of your training time.

Remember that this plan is based on three weeks of active training, followed by a week of rest, then another three weeks of training and a week of rest. Make sure that when you start each new three-week training period, you do so from the time you finished the last three-week program. If, for example, you finished your last three-week period with a major workout

40-minute program time, that's the starting point. You DO NOT start over again and of course this is still subject to a maximum of 75 minutes per session in total.

This program will certainly improve your fitness levels simply because you are exercising regularly.

In terms of technique, however, improvements may not be as easy to recognize by yourself, so it's a good idea to ask for help from others who can give you an impartial assessment of how much you've improved, and what you still have to do in technical terms.

If you have a friend who is a strong swimmer, or perhaps someone who is a recognized expert, such as a lifeguard, would be a good person to ask for help.

Otherwise, your local pool may have a swim coach and, in that case, you could book a few professional training sessions as a way to identify and then "eliminate" any technical defect or weakness.

Remember that the idea of improving

your technique is not to become an international class swimmer! However, without good technique you won't get the maximum benefits in terms of fitness either, so don't neglect the technical aspect of swimming.

Just do this... Jump!

Jumping is another excellent form of aerobic exercise that you can do literally anytime, anywhere.

It helps improve both the heart and lungs, as well as improve flexibility, coordination, and, of course, fitness.

Jumping may seem like an easy option at first glance, but you may find that it can be much more difficult than you think if you decide to keep jumping for a certain period of time. Remember that boxers use skipping as an integral part of their training programs between games, and they are not generally known for doing things the easy way, so you should tell them how effective skipping is as a form of training exercise.

Jumping also represents high-intensity training, as indicated by the fact that twenty minutes of jumping burn 250 kilocalories of energy. It is ideal to help shape and tone the lower body, especially the calves, hips, thighs and buttocks.

In fact, jumping is directly comparable to running at 12 km/h in terms of the energy being burned, but because it is an activity that involves a lower level of impact than running, it is much softer on joints and less likely to cause injuries than hitting sidewalks or using a running machine.

However, jumping obviously involves jumping up and down and therefore some consequences have to be taken into account. Therefore, it is necessary to take some basic and sensible precautions.

For example, you must make sure you have a rope that is the correct length for your height.

To test this, stand on the rope at the midpoint and lift the handles at each end. If the rope is of the correct length, then the point where the rope and handles meet should be at a level with the armpits.

If it's too short, it needs a longer rope. However, if it is too long, all you need to do is artificially shorten it by tying knots in the rope as close to the handles as possible. This is a good idea if more than one person uses the same rope.

When you're jumping, you can also reduce the potentially adverse effects of "landing" impact by wearing shoes with padded soles, and trying to jump on surfaces that have something to "give way" on them.

For example, jumping on a wooden floor (which has some "flex") will be better than jumping on a tile or concrete floor.

For most of us, the last time we skipped was probably many years ago, so in case you've forgotten, here are the basics of how to jump to get the maximum benefits from exercise:

- Stand up but relax while doing so, and try to breathe normally.

- Keep your elbows at waist level, but your arms should extend sideways at an angle of about 90 degrees to your body.

- You need to perfect a circular movement of the wrist to rotate the jump rope.

- Grasp the handles of the rope without squeezing them and use your thumbs and index fingers as a means of controlling the rope.

- Jump off the balls of your feet and try to cushion your landing (which should be back on the balls of your feet) by flexing your knees.

This isn't the Olympic high jump competition! You just need to jump high enough to allow the rope to pass under your feet. If you can do this successfully, then doing about 60 laps per minute (i.e. one per second) should be an achievable initial goal.

It will take a bit of practice, but once you have mastered these basic concepts, then you may want to start doing some tricks and jumping 'acrobatics', both as a way to make your session a little more interesting and also to show off your newfound talents!

Believe it or not, according to the International Rope Jumping Federation website, there are over a hundred simple rope tricks you can learn, including favorites such as the "double bounce," the "skier," and the "bell:

Skipping is a very simple but extremely effective form of exercise that anyone can do anywhere. Don't underestimate your benefits just because you haven't jumped on a rope once since the day you left school!

Stretching, folding and toning

So far, all the exercise formats we've considered have focused on the aerobic side of exercising, doing activities that will burn energy while working the heart and lungs a little harder.

However, not all exercise is necessarily aerobic, as there are many exercises that focus more on toning and shaping the body, while increasing things like flexibility and flexibility.

Such exercises are no less beneficial than the aerobic exercises we've seen so far, and you may be surprised at how many ways it's possible to practice these exercises without making too much obvious effort.

Let us now begin to examine some of these exercises.

Let's start with the... Yoga

Yoga has been practiced around the world for about 5,000 years, and is an active exercise that essentially consists of a combination of positions, postures and postures. Taken together, they will improve your strength and flexibility while serving to lower stress levels while calming your "inner self.

Although for the purposes of this book we are focusing on yoga as a form of exercise, yoga is, in fact, much more than that. It is a complete way of life, bringing together the spirit, mind and body of man in a unified system of beliefs and actions.

There are several types or branches of yoga, with the exercises we are going to see (known as 'Asanas') being part of the yogic branch called Hatha Yoga (which means forced yoga) which is especially popular in the West.

Yogic exercises are composed of many asanas, all of which have varying degrees of difficulty in physical terms. However, the degree of physical difficulty is only part of the story, because many yogic postures focus less on the physical nature of the postulation in question, and much more on the spiritual aspect.

For example, the pose or position that would appear to be the least physically demanding is the 'shava-asana' or corpse pose. This requires the student to lie on his or her back, with hands at his or her sides.

In physical terms it couldn't be easier,

but the point is that what you're really trying to do is make the whole body and mind totally still and relaxed. Without that total stillness, the 'shave-asana' is not really complete, according to yogic thought.

While keeping your body completely still may not be so difficult, doing the same with your mind is much more difficult, to the point that many people would find everything but impossible. Trying the 'shava-asna' is therefore extremely easy, but achieving it properly is definitely not so.

Unusual exercises you've never thought about

As previously suggested, focusing on toning the body is as important as burning energy through aerobic exercise.

However, there are several parts of the body that most of us never consider to be in need of exercise.

Your whole body needs exercise if the various parts of your body are to remain in perfect condition.

In this section, I'm going to look at some of the body parts that are most often neglected, and how you can exercise them using simple, direct everyday activities.

> ***Exercise the face***

It is almost certain that your face is a part of your body that you have never considered exercising.

But you do need it, especially if you want to open up your features, remove skin lines and get a clearer, younger expression.

Exercising the face is about using the facial muscles that are less used in daily life, because this strengthens these muscles and therefore the face becomes more flexible and expressive.

Before starting these exercises, you should take a good, long look in the mirror to decide which exercises you should focus on personally. If, for example, you are naturally a frown, then don't bother with the frowning exercise. Instead, focus on smiling or winking, for example.

Here are four extremely easy and

painless facial exercises that you can start doing right now:

Smiling: Paraphrasing a phrase from Casablanca, "You know how to smile, don't you?". If not, here's how to do it to get the most out of smiling.

With your head in an upright but relaxed posture, squeeze your cheeks up while extending your lips over your teeth at the same time.

Hold the position for a few seconds, then relax and repeat the process. Do this 15 to 20 times per session, and try to do it at least once a day.

Try to smile at other people more often as well. You may be surprised at how much better it makes you feel spiritually, and the answers you get will more than justify the small effort involved.

Frowning: In this exercise, you start with your head straight but relaxed, only this time you'll tighten your forehead muscles and lower your eyebrows as you do so. Hold the resulting frown for a few seconds and then release it, and do the exercise 15-20 times per session.

This is an exercise that should only be done in moderation, as overuse of these muscles by doing this exercise too regularly or can often lead to the development of unwanted facial lines and wrinkles.

Yawing: With the head in the (already) traditional vertical and relaxed position, turn the head slightly to one side so that one eye is pushed slightly forward. Close the most prominent eye and keep it closed for a second or two. Open the eye again and repeat the operation 15 to 20 times with the same eye.

Then, turn your head to the other side so that the opposite eye is in the foreground, and repeat the entire process with that eye.

Again, you probably don't want to exaggerate in this particular exercise, as doing so can lead to the formation (or acceleration) of fine creases and wrinkles in the corners of the eyes that are commonly referred to as "laugh lines.

Also, I would recommend that this is an exercise that is done in a private place, because doing this in public or with people you don't know around you could give them a completely wrong idea.

Tongue twitches: This is an exercise that you should only do privately or with people you know. While winking at strangers could get you a lot of unwanted attention, it's much more likely to slap you in the face or punch you in the nose, so be careful where and when you decide to do this exercise!

Start from the relaxed but upright position of the head and purses the lips slightly. Then, take your tongue out of your mouth (yes, just like when you were a child) and then remove it.

Assuming that you don't regularly walk pulling your tongue towards people, this is an action that the muscles in the back of your tongue will rarely undertake. While your tongue is used to moving up and down and side-to-side inside your mouth while you're eating or talking, this "back to front push" is using the muscles in a way they're not used to.

Repeat this exercise 15-20 times per session.

> ***Foot and leg exercises***

If you have traveled on a long-haul flight in recent times, you probably know that many of the major airlines are demonstrating safety.

videos that emphasize the importance of moving your feet and legs during flight. This is to counteract the increased risk of deep vein thrombosis that can cause you to spend several hours in a pressurized cabin.

Similarly, more and more people spend most of their working day sitting and are therefore not using their legs as much as they should.

Sometimes they go to the bathroom and maybe walk outside the office for lunch, so they're not totally idle, but they're almost certainly not using their leg and lower back muscles as much as they should.

Like the videos you see on airplanes, I'm going to show you several ways you can make your muscles work even when you're sitting.

Crossing legs: This exercise is exactly what it looks like, but as safety videos on the plane suggest, even moving your legs and feet while sitting can stimulate blood flow and muscle activity in your legs.

Therefore, it is simply a matter of sitting in your chair, relaxing and then crossing one leg up and over the top of the other. Hold that end position for less than a second - in this case, it is the action and movement that is important, not the end position - and then return to the original relaxed position.

Do the same 15-20 times and then repeat the actions for the other leg.

- Swinging: This exercise is almost an extension of the crossing movement we used in the last one.

After crossing your legs, you should swing the foot at the top forward and then back again in a pendulum motion.

This causes the muscles in the back of the legs to contract and expand in the effort to elevate the foot, and this stimulates the muscles and increases blood flow in the legs.

As always, repeat 15 to 20 times for each leg, and try not to do so in an environment where you may run the risk of kicking others while exercising.

The swivel: This is easy, but effective for keeping your calves and ankles, in particular, in good shape.

You can also do it sitting in your chair or on the floor of your house, with your legs stretched out in front of you.

All you have to do is turn your feet at the ankles so that the toes of both feet are pointing at each other, and then turn back again so that the heels do the same. Repeat this as many times as you want (at least 20 would be good) and use this exercise whenever you have been sitting for long periods as a means of "cooling" your legs.

Tip, touch: Even just tapping your toes on the floor will keep your feet, ankles and calves active and ensure that your muscles are stimulated to stimulate blood flow in the lower legs.

Whether you're wearing shoes in the office or sitting at home barefoot, simply lift your left toes off the floor and strike them again two or three times. Rest for a moment - you shouldn't need much time, as this is not strenuous - and then repeat. Do this 15 to 20 times with the same foot and then repeat the exercise with the opposite foot.

This is an exercise that is best done with music!

➤ *Back and Buttock Exercises*

Change and lift: This is an exercise you can do to strengthen the muscles of your lower back and buttocks (in particular) while sitting. Therefore, this is something that can be done even while you are at work, although given the nature of the "lifting" element of the exercise, I would not really recommend that you do this while talking to other people in the office, for example. I could make them think there's something wrong with you.

However, this is a great exercise to reduce any stiffness or pain that may result from sitting in the same position for an extended period of time, and it also strengthens those muscles.

While in your chair, relax and then squeeze the muscle in one buttock and hold it for a couple of seconds, lifting it slightly as you do so.

Relax and then repeat. Do this 15 to 20 times per buttock.

Hip Swing: This is a great exercise to do if you are standing for any period of time, as it relieves tension in your legs and stimulates

the blood flow through the entire lower part of your body. It also helps to avoid the lower back pain that afflicts some people if they are forced to stand for a long time.

While standing, let your right knee relax and soften, while at the same time pushing your left hip to one side. Pull the hip back and repeat the same action 15-20 times.

After that, allow your left knee to bend and relax, and force your right hip out in the same way.

- Lifting: Grab a bag - a plastic bag from the supermarket, or anything else that has adequate handles to lift it will do the trick.

Put some weight into the bag - again, it's pretty irrelevant exactly what it is, as long as it weighs at least a few kilos (water bottles are ideal for this, because you know that a one liter bottle weighs almost exactly one kilo).

Holding your right arm down to one

side, bend your knees until you can reach the bag on the floor and then lift it up by stretching your knees up. Lift until your legs are straight again, hold the "up" position for a few seconds and then put the bag back on the floor by bending your knees one more time.

Repeat 15 times on one side of your body and then repeat on the opposite side.

When done correctly, i.e. bending your knees and not from your back, this exercise is excellent for strengthening the lower back, buttocks and hips, but also helps keep your arms and thighs in good shape.

- Make us shrug our shoulders: This is an exercise that not only helps keep the lower back strong, but is also an effective way to release the tension that can build up in the shoulders and neck. It will help you keep your arms and shoulder muscles toned and fit at the same time.

It can also be done standing or sitting.

Wherever you are, simply lift your shoulders toward your ears with the classic shrugging motion, then lift your forearms to a position where they are parallel to the ground and turn your palms outward.

Finally, tilt your head to one side and turn it slightly from your neck, then hold that final position for a few seconds. Go back to the beginning and do it all over again, but this time, tilt your head to the opposite side before turning.

Conclusion

Very few people are completely unaware of the fact that exercise is good for them.

The problem is that, for many people, even when they know this, the idea of having to join a gym and actually go through the physical shredder in an effort to get in shape is totally unpleasant.

Therefore, they chose to ignore the fact that their body condition is deteriorating and move on with their lives in exactly the same way they did before, unless some event occurs that causes them to change.

The point I hope you appreciate now after reading this book is that you don't have to wait until you have to start exercising before taking any action. There are literally dozens of opportunities to work some part of your body every day of your life, and all you need to do to start exercising is to recognize these opportunities.

Nor should exercise automatically equate with hard work, monotony, and pain.

As you have seen, simple activities such as walking and climbing stairs can be integrated into your daily life quickly and almost perfectly, but the benefits of these two activities can be enormous.

The bottom line is that there's no excuse not to start exercising right now, and everything you need to know to do it is contained in this book.

There's no better time to start doing regular exercise than this second, so put on your shoes, go for a long walk, and take the time to think about all the other ways you're going to make exercise an integral part of your life from now on.

Just remember that everything will not happen overnight and that it will take time before you see a change in your life for the better.

Now yes, I wish you the best in your results, and remember, everything is practical; theory without action is of no use to you. It brings everything you learn into real life.

A big hug, your friend, Jessy!

By the way, when you achieve your results little by little, I highly recommend you, if you want to learn much more about methods of losing weight, my book, on "HOW TO MAKE THE CETOGENIC DIET WITHOUT STOP EATING", is a book that I am sure will help you a lot on your way to "good health". Without further ado, you can find it in the Amazon search engine, like: "How to do the ketogenic diet without stopping eating" or looking for my name, like: "Jessy M. Brown"... Once again I wish you success in your results!